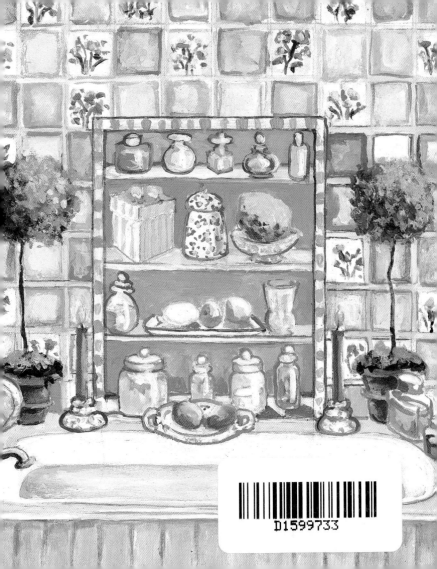

In memory of Grandma Rosey,
who soaked to soothe and heal

Illustrator and painter Katharine Barnwell
studied at Pratt Institute, The Art Students
League, and under the tutelage of Nerina Simi
in Florence, Italy. Her work includes *Seeds
from a Secret Garden* and *Sow the Seeds of Love*,
both published by Peter Pauper Press.

~ The ~
Enchanted Bath

Bath Rituals and Recipes

By Susan Hayden

Illustrated by Katharine Barnwell

Designed by Mullen & Katz

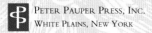

PETER PAUPER PRESS, INC.
WHITE PLAINS, NEW YORK

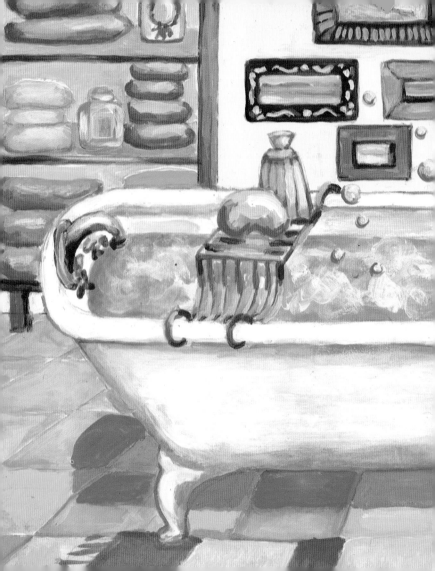

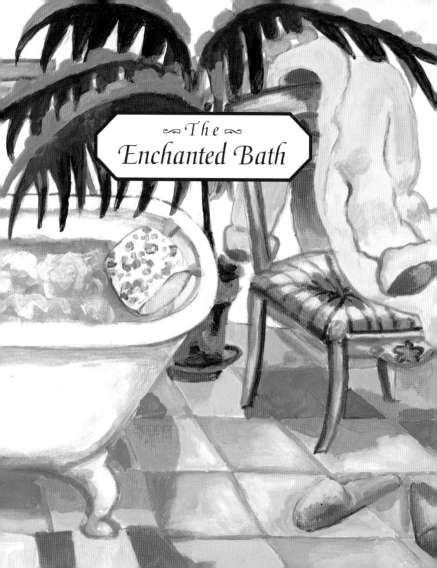

The Enchanted Bath

Contents

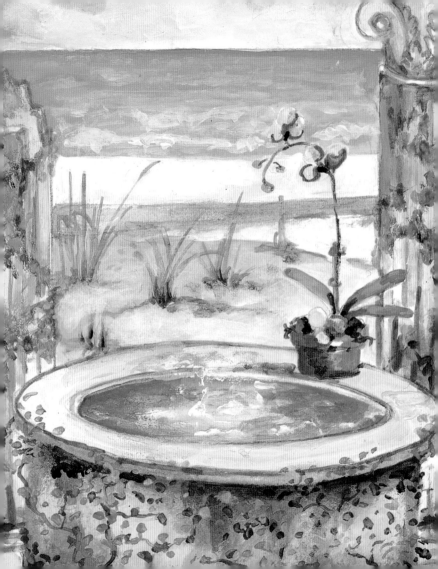

∾ The ∾
Original Home

You hear the sound of water
and you know where you want to be.

Rumi

*I*n today's world, it is very difficult to set aside the time to indulge in a few moments of luxury. We forget that by simply washing away the pressures of daily life we can replenish and reinforce our well-being. The bath is a celebration of the whole self. It is a reward to the body, mind, and soul. The bath helps to nurture, balance, and release energy. It is one place in your home that you can go to, again and again, to attain inner tranquillity.

A bath relaxes the mind and body and connects us to an ancient ritual. Water is pure, rejuvenating therapy, tried and true.

To honor our bodies and ourselves with fragrant oils of flowers and herbs is to intertwine with nature. In a sanctuary of scent and warm water, we can breathe deeply, rejoice, and feel the wholeness of life.

We soak and bathe as a ritual of remembrance. We burn candles and create our own private retreat, linked with what is holy and enchanting. Water is the great beginning, the sea of life, our first dwelling place. When we take a bath, we are reminded of where we came from, and where we want to return. It is the original home.

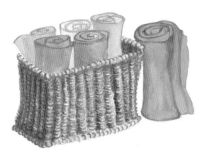

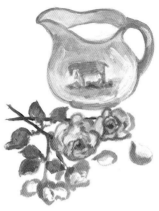

Aromatherapy can be considered a healing art. However, the material in this book is not intended to take the place of diagnosis and treatment by a qualified medical practitioner. All recommendations are believed to be effective, yet the actual use of essential oils by others is beyond the author's control. Therefore, no expressed or implied guarantee can be given as to the effects of the use of essential oils.

Use only stainless steel, glass, or ceramic containers when mixing essential oils, so as not to alter their chemical properties.

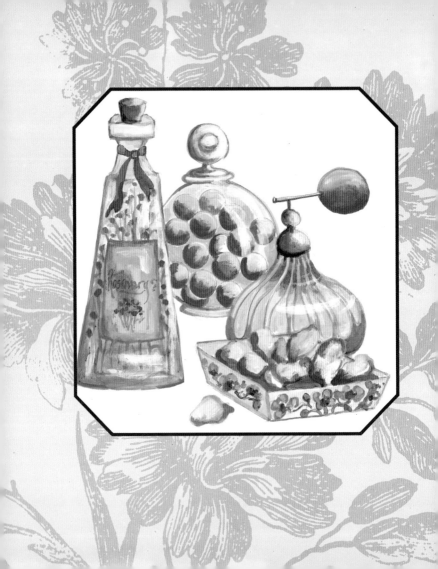

Temperatures
of the Bath

Cool
65–80 degrees F.

Tepid
80–92 degrees F.

Neutral to Warm
92–98 degrees F.

Hot
98–104 degrees F.

Very Hot (dangerous)
104–115 degrees F.

Remedy
of the Sages

Therapeutic Bathing
in Ancient Times

*The springs . . .
to bathe in them gives new life;
to drink them cures every bodily ill.*

Cherokee Wisdom

*E*arly civilizations practiced what we now refer to as holistic medicine. The mind, body, and spirit were all considered in the healing process. Health was aligned with nature. Massage, aromatherapy, herbology, and the bath were common treatments. Water was the remedy of the sages.

The oldest known medical document, the Ayurveda of India, written in Sanskrit, prescribed the blending of herbs and warm oils in bath form. Designed to prevent aging and immortality, this treatment was originally reserved for king and queens. Now you can treat yourself royally too!

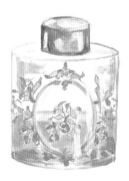

Parvati's Indian Summer Soak
for Unwinding

Parvati is the Hindu goddess of the mountains,
the daughter of the Himalayas. She is known as the ruler of
nature spirits.

THE BOTANICALS

5 drops jasmine essential oil
5 drops sandalwood essential oil
2 teaspoons sulfated castor oil

Draw a warm bath. In a bowl, blend essential oils and
castor oil. Add to bath water, mixing with your hands. Soak
for 20-30 minutes.

THE MOOD

Begin by playing Indian or Near Eastern stringed instru-
ments like the sitar or the tambura. Burn sweetly-scented
patchouli incense or a brown candle (Parvati's sacred color).
Sip from a glass of hot ginger tea. When you finish bathing,
wrap yourself in a colorful sarong and relax.

The Egyptians cleansed their spirits through bathing as far back as 4000 B.C. They revered water as a divine substance that embodied magical properties.

Greeks and Romans followed suit, though in ancient Rome only the wealthiest of people could afford bathrooms of their own. Majestic bathing halls were soon created in every town for public use. Floors, columns, and seats were made of marble. Walls were inlaid with precious gems, and ceilings were often hand-painted. These bathhouses became centers for cultural activities, housing art galleries, lecture halls, and massage rooms. The baths of Caracalla could hold up to 1,600 bathers at a time; it was a grand setting for social gatherings and worldly meetings.

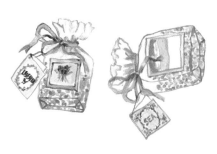

Hygieia's Love-Thy-Body Bath

For Physical Self-Esteem

Hygieia, the goddess of health, was the offspring of Asclepius, the god of healing.

THE BOTANICALS

3 drops rosemary essential oil
2 drops ylang-ylang essential oil
1 drop patchouli essential oil
1 drop peppermint essential oil
2 teaspoons sulfated castor oil

Fill your bathtub with warm to hot water. In a bowl blend essential oils with castor oil. Pour in tub and mix thoroughly with your hands. Bathe for 20 minutes.

THE MOOD

A beautiful body is not created by diet and exercise alone. It involves one's self-perception. Trust your intuition and avoid following external ideas of how you should look. Accept yourself for who you are. Light silver candles to remove negativity. Inhale deeply and then exhale, releasing all thoughts about your physical being that are not positive. Remember, you're worth it!

Women
a n d *Water*

History and Myths of
Females and the Bath

*Water is the most healing of all
remedies, and the best of all cosmetics.*
Old Arabian Proverb

Women have always been linked to water, both historically and mythologically. Queen Cleopatra bathed in milk, water, and rose petals in preparation to attract Mark Antony. It worked! Queen Elizabeth of Hungary took a bath in rosemary water, then drank it and massaged it into her paralyzed joints, curing herself and winning the heart of a much younger man.

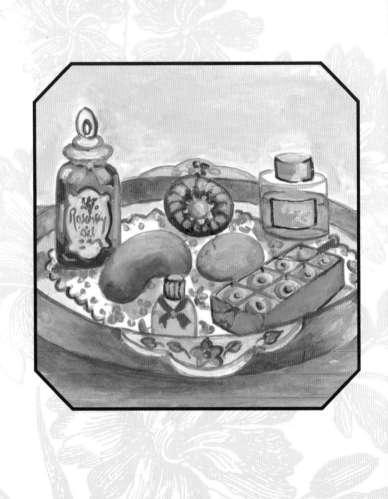

French Impressionist painters like Renoir and Cézanne used the bathing female as a recurring motif in their work. Angelic and sublime, these beauties were painted to look spiritually cleansed and at peace. Women and water was also an enduring theme for the Pre-Raphaelites.

Aphrodite, Greek goddess of love, whose name is derived from the word *aphros*, meaning sea-foam, was said to have sprung from the ocean before floating to Cyprus. She is identified by the Romans with Venus, the goddess of fertility and beauty, who emerged from the sea, where she was presented with a single red rose.

And then there is the mermaid. She descended from folklore that connected goddesses with the sea, the universal womb. Stories of fish-deities and sea-geishas were told by fishermen from every land. Idealized as beautiful, uninhibited, and dangerous water creatures, they were thought to rule with hypnotic charm. The most legendary mermaid was Melusine. After marrying a mortal who built her a castle, she would spend one day a week spread out in her bath, in the strictest of privacy, for that is when her tail would appear.

Cleopatra's Bath of Roses
To Awaken the Senses

Cleopatra was a flamboyant and earthy queen who carpeted her floor with petals of roses and used their essential oil to entice her man. Cleopatra wasn't the only one to bathe in milk, but she may have been the first. Do you think she knew that roses mean confidence?

THE BOTANICALS

6-10 drops rose essential oil
1/4-1/2 cup goat's milk

In a small bowl, mix rose essential oil into the goat's milk. Add to a hot bath. Sprinkle with fresh rose petals. Soak for at least 20 minutes.

THE MOOD

Imagine yourself in ancient Egypt, circa 45 B.C., when it was the wealthiest kingdom in the Mediterranean. Why not use rose petals like those you just threw in the hot bath to cover your floor, too? Burn orange candles, to stimulate and energize, and be sure to turn out all the lights. To honor the queen, have your flashiest bathrobe ready to slip into when you finish soaking in the milk bath. Cleopatra loved silk, and her favorite colors were purple and gold.

Aphrodite's Conjuring Waters

For Pure Pleasure

The Greeks worshipped Aphrodite. She was their feminine ideal and one of the Twelve Great Olympians, and was known as "Queen of the Sea."

THE BOTANICALS

4 drops ginger essential oil
4 drops sandalwood essential oil
4 drops vanilla essential oil
4 drops ylang-ylang essential oil
1 tablespoon sulfated castor oil

In a bowl, mix essential oils with castor oil. Pour into hot bath water, blending with your hands. Soak 20–30 minutes.

THE MOOD

Picture an idyllic sunbathed island in the Aegean Sea. Get some nisiotika (Greek Island) music by Yianni Parios, or classic bouzouki. Light a red candle, to attract the influence of Aphrodite. Let the moonlight shine through the window and imagine three sailors are doing the hasapiko (Greek folk/napkin dance) just for you.

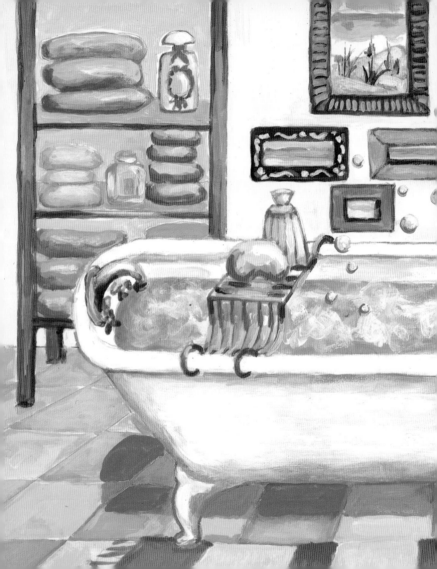

❧ The ❧
Fragrant Soul

*Aromatherapy
and Essential Oils*

*He is happiest who hath power to
gather wisdom from a flower.*

Mary Howitt, ca. 1825

Aromatherapy. The word brings to mind scent and healing. It is an ancient practice, a science, and an art. Naturally distilled essences are extracted from plants and used for one's physical, mental, and emotional well-being. Called essential oils, they are said to possess healing properties for the mind, body, and spirit. Tiny droplets contained in fruit, leaves, bark, stems, roots, and flowers are responsible for each botanical's individual smell.

In many cultures, healing with plants and their essential oils was a part of everyday life. Aromatics were used for ceremonies, art, beauty, and medicinal purposes. Incense was the original perfume. It was believed that burning incense was a link to one's ancestors, and a way to connect with universal energy.

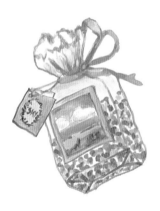

The Egyptians were among the first to experiment with aromatherapy. Incense was burned at all times in their temples, to inspire inner transformation and heighten the spiritual experience. Herbal and floral essences were used to anoint the skin and were utilized in the bath for health, physical attractiveness, and protection.

The historic Vedic texts of India specifically ascribe various therapeutic and medicinal powers to aromatic plants. The practice of perfumery was frequently mentioned in early Sanskrit literature.

The use of botanicals can be found in China as far back as the Shang Dynasty (1600 to 1100 B.C.). Centuries later in Japan, Samurai warriors used incense to scent their helmets and armor in preparation for battle. The Greeks attributed divine origin to sweet smells. Gods supposedly dropped down to earth on clouds that were scented, in robes soaked with fragrant essences. The bathhouses of both Greece and Rome used essential oils for massage, bathing, and overall health purposes.

Aromatherapy's modern renaissance began in the 1920s, when René-Maurice Gattefosse, a French chemist and perfumer, was experimenting with fragrance in his lab and burned his hand. He plunged it into the liquid closest to him, a tub of lavender oil; his hand healed quickly and without a scar! From then on, he dedicated his life to researching the therapeutic value of essential oils, thus coining the term aromatherapy.

Whether inhaled or absorbed through the skin, each essential oil carries its own benefit to which the body and mind will respond. When different oils from the same therapeutic category are blended, they can create synergy. This means that the individual oils will usually complement each other when combined, enhancing the treatment.

Essential oils should never be applied directly to the skin by themselves, for they will irritate it. Carrier oils are necessary to transport the substances. Unprocessed, organic, and cold-pressed oils are preferable; they are pressed from the seed, nut, or fruit, with no chemical solvents added to them. Best for the bath is sulfated castor oil. It is the only carrier oil that is dispersible in water and will not leave a residue.

The power of smell is immeasurable. A scent can work on a subconscious level to balance, harmonize, calm, relax, energize, or stimulate. Aromatherapy connects us with our memories and links us to nature, while activating our bodies' own healing energies.

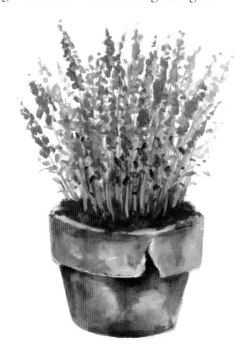

Sleepytime Soak
For the Sweetest of Dreams

Ancient cultures massaged chamomile oil into the skin to alleviate aches and pain, relieve muscle soreness, and cool fever. Its subtle action is said to eliminate anxiety, stabilize stress levels, and calm the spirit.

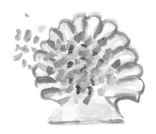

THE BOTANICALS

1/2 cup Dead Sea salts
4 drops chamomile essential oil
2 drops marjoram essential oil
2 drops ylang-ylang essential oil
1 drop basil essential oil
2 chamomile tea bags

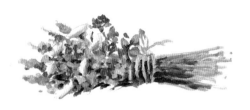

Boil two cups of water to make some chamomile tea, leaving tea bags in the cup until you are ready to bathe. Mix bath salt and oils in a bowl and pour into a full warm or hot bath. Disperse well, blending with your hands.

THE MOOD

Set a tranquil tone. Light blue candles; they soothe, relax, and create serenity. Burn some sandalwood incense. Dim the lights. Play uplifting music, such as Vivaldi's "The Four Seasons." Place warm drained chamomile tea bags over your closed eyes, and sip from your cup. Think of the ocean at low tide, remnants of slow waves at your feet. Now drift . . .

Only Hearts Immersion

To Deepen Feelings

Medieval Europeans believed lavender to be the herb of love. It promotes deep relaxation and has a balancing effect on the skin.

THE BOTANICALS

3 drops lavender essential oil
3 drops ylang-ylang essential oil
2 drops coriander essential oil
1 drop neroli essential oil
2 teaspoons sulfated castor oil

In a bowl, mix essential oils with castor oil; add to hot water and swish. Bathe for 20–30 minutes.

THE MOOD

This bath brings to mind Venus, the Roman goddess of love and beauty. Her sacred candle color is pink; light just one candle. Stare into the candle and think of who or what needs more care of the heart.

Scentuality

===

How to Make
Your Environment Fragrant
with Essential Oils

1 drop on a love letter

1 drop on a lace hankie

2 drops on a small cloth,
thrown into the dryer to scent your laundry

3 drops on someone else's pillow

4 drops on a light bulb,
for perfumed air

6 drops mixed into 1 ounce of
unscented cream, for fragrant skin

12 drops mixed into 1 ounce of
vegetable oil, for a sensual massage

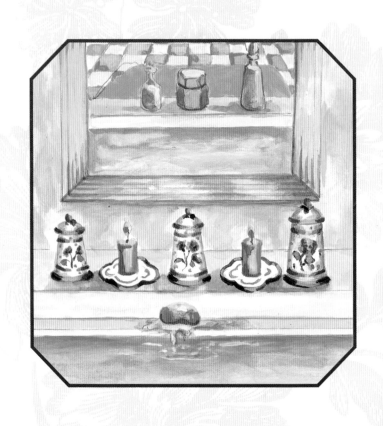

Sacred Fires

────────

Creating Ambiance and
Healing Meditations
with Candles

*We are born into
the world of nature; our second birth
is into the world of spirit.*
Bhagavad-Gita

Atmosphere is the great beginning. Setting the tone is the first step. Why not create a room for the bath that is your personal sanctuary of nourishment and harmony? If this does not seem possible because you share the space with others, there's hope! Fill a basket with scented candles, a natural fiber washcloth, recordings of your favorite music, a framed picture of someone you love or a place that holds special memories, a book of affirmations, and a variety of essential oils. Keep it hidden in a drawer, ready and waiting to give your body and spirit the healing retreat you are worthy of.

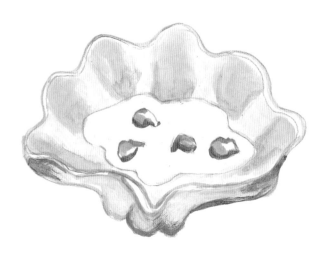

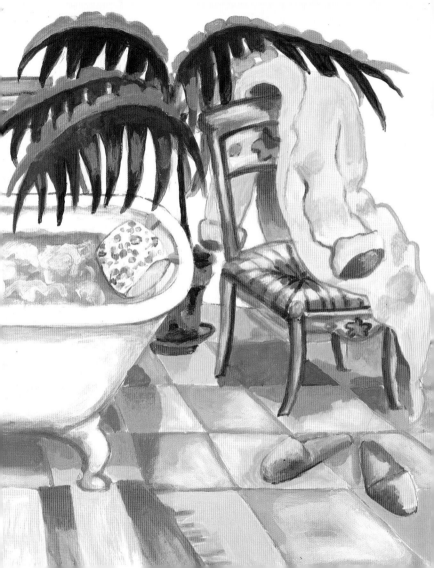

Natural Woman Bubble Bath
To Connect with All Things Elemental

Mandarin oil has been used to alleviate fatigue, stress, and restlessness. It helps to uplift the spirit and get back to the true you.

THE BOTANICALS

4 drops mandarin essential oil
4 drops lavender essential oil
1 cup unscented bubble bath
1/4 cup glycerin

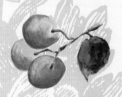

In a bowl, mix bubble bath and glycerin. Add essential oils and stir to blend. Pour into a warm or hot bath, blending mixture into water with your hands. Light green candles, the color of nature.

THE MOOD

You've been hiking for hours. Now, as the sun casts a rich alpenglow on the granite ridge above, you immerse yourself into the warm waters of a natural hot spring. Your aches and pains dissolve. A feeling of wondrous relaxation takes their place. Close your eyes; breathe deeply. Let the earth-mother in you soar!

THE MEDITATION

*Speak to the earth
and it shall teach thee.*

Job 12:8

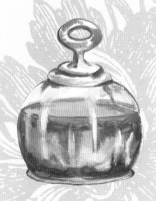

$\mathcal{L}$ighting candles was once a highly symbolic gesture, linked to the preservation of the soul. The mellow glow of a candle creates an immediate aura of white light that radiates throughout the room. The element of fire creates light in darkness, and signifies transformation.

The candle is the image of humanity; its wax corresponds to the physical body, its wick to the mind, its flame to the spirit or soul. Candles are key to any ceremony, meditation, or ritual. Rituals speak to the heart and to the soul. They make everyday life more holy and enriching.

Clear the mind by lighting a candle, reclining in a hot bath full of essential oils, and gazing into a flame. It is an ancient way to feel rooted, to come home, back to your authentic self.

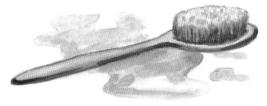

Scents and Sensibility Dip
For Self-Affirmation and Rejuvenation

Bergamot gives Earl Grey tea its distinctive flavor. Its oil evokes feelings of happiness and equalizes emotions. Petitgrain is from the orange flower. Its essential oil comes from behind the stem. This bath is good for getting back onto the purposeful path.

THE BOTANICALS

4 drops bergamot essential oil
4 drops petitgrain essential oil
2 teaspoons sulfated castor oil

In a cup, combine castor oil with essential oils by stirring. Draw a warm bath and blend mixture in with your hands.

THE MOOD AND THE MEDITATION

This is a celebration of the powerful life force that is within you. It may be invisible, but it is boundless. White candles everywhere symbolize innocence and peace. Play Chopin, perhaps "Ballade No. 1 in G Minor." Put tulips, also white, in a jelly jar. This is the perfect time to reassess your goals and affirm the path you are on. Pick one candle to gaze into and say this meditation aloud, or silently, to yourself:

I follow my energy and purpose, trust in the life force, and believe that the universe will take care of me.

*I*f you are lighting a candle for a reason other than ambiance, the color should be selected carefully, according to your purpose. Each color has meaning and possesses a different vibration that attracts specific influences. Every candle color corresponds to a mythological goddess:

Yellow: For charm, confidence, attraction, and persuasion. Sacred color of Amaterasu-O-Mi-Kami, the Japanese sun goddess.

Orange: To stimulate and energize. One of the sacred colors of Demeter, the goddess of agriculture in Greek mythology.

Gold: To attract cosmic influences. Sacred color of Fortuna, Roman goddess of happiness and good fortune.

White: For healing, inner peace, and spiritual strength. Sacred color of Flora, Roman goddess of flowers.

Silver: To encourage stability. Sacred color of Kilya, Inca moon goddess.

Red: For fertility, passion, love, and magnetism. Sacred color of Aphrodite.

Purple: For psychic energy, healing, success, power, and independence. Sacred color of Athena, Greek goddess of wisdom and the arts.

Pink: For love and friendship. Sacred color of Benten, Japanese love goddess of femininity, music, literature, and the sea.

Green: For good luck, fertility, prosperity, and rejuvenation. Sacred color of Kuan Yin, the Chinese goddess of childbirth and compassion.

Blue: For honor and loyalty, truth, tranquillity, wisdom, and peace. Sacred color of Hathor, Egyptian goddess of beauty and the heavens.

Brown: To improve powers of concentration and protection. Sacred color of Parvati, Hindu goddess of the mountains.

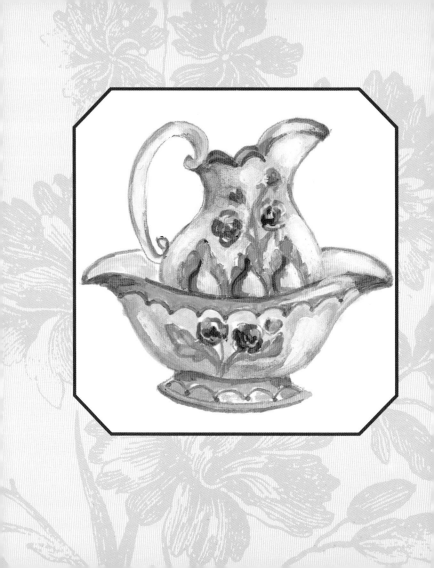

Beauty Takes
a Bath

*The Six Steps to
Complexion Care*

*I adore simple pleasures. They are the
last refuge of the complex.*

Oscar Wilde

There's not a better time to treat your face with tender care than before, during, and after the bath. Here are six simple steps and some all-natural, homemade recipes. Each mixture includes essential oils or herbs, which restore balance and harmony and promote the health of your body and mind. If this sensible regimen is followed consistently, a peaches and cream complexion will be yours.

Step One

CLEANSING

Cleansers remove impurities from the skin. Cleanse once in the morning and again before bedtime.

Step Two

EXFOLIATION

A facial scrub, when gently applied, will slough off dead surface skin, expose fresh skin, boost circulation, and give you a healthy glow. Exfoliate 1–3 times a week. Not for sensitive skin.

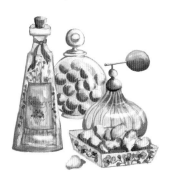

Greenhouse Savory Scrub

Geranium oil is considered the first-aid kit of essential oils, with its antiseptic and regenerative qualities. Lavender oil boosts the immune system and stimulates new cell growth. This scrub will give your skin a youthful freshness and vitality.

THE BOTANICALS

1 teaspoon almond meal or blue cornmeal
1 teaspoon honey
1 drop geranium essential oil
1 drop lavender essential oil

Place all ingredients in blender. Make a paste in your palm. Massage over skin for one minute. Rinse thoroughly.

Step Three

TONING

Toners remove residues left on the skin by a cleanser, mask, or scrub. Toners improve the general health and appearance of the skin, and prepare your face to absorb a moisturizer. Tone twice a day.

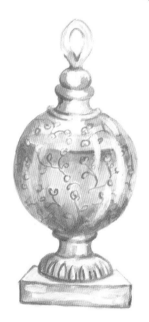

Sacred Grove Soothing Toner

The Assyrians believed that the secret names of the gods were written on the sacred cedar. Cedarwood is a calming oil that stabilizes energy imbalances and normalizes the skin.

Ylang-Ylang oil was used in the Victorian era as part of a hair growth preparation. It inspires creativity and wards off premature aging by releasing tension in the face.

THE BOTANICALS

2 ounces witch hazel
1 tablespoon aloe vera
5 drops cedarwood essential oil
3 drops lemon essential oil
1 drop ylang-ylang essential oil

Combine ingredients. Shake well before using.

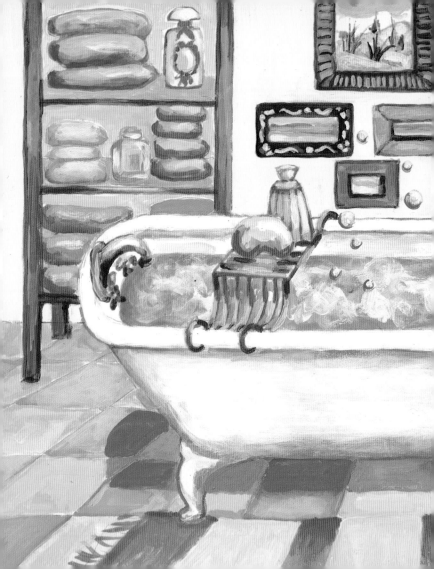

Step Four

MOISTURIZING

Moisturizers create a protective barrier between your skin and the atmosphere, plump up surface skin, prevent moisture loss, and give a soft, smooth appearance. Apply after cleaning and toning, twice a day.

Step Five

STEAMING

Steaming with essential oils will deeply clean your pores, moisturize your skin, and improve circulation to your face. Steam once or twice a week.

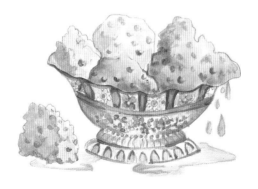

Herbs du Jour Garden Steam

Eucalyptus restores balance, improves concentration, and is believed to increase intellectual capacity. It also relieves stress and encourages alertness. This herbal mini-sauna's strong anti-bacterial action will promote the regeneration of skin tissue and will help eliminate excess oil.

THE BOTANICALS

3 cups spring water
1 drop eucalyptus essential oil
1 drop lavender essential oil
1 drop rosemary essential oil

Boil water and wait until it cools to about 100 degrees F. Pour it into a bowl, add essential oils, and set bowl in a place where you are comfortable. Cover the back of your head with a towel, tucking the ends around your head so that the towel encloses both your head and the bowl. Hold your head one foot away from water. Make sure steam is not so hot as to be uncomfortable. Keep your eyes closed and stay in steam for a few minutes; then come out to cool your face. Repeat.

Step Six

MASKS

A moisturizing mask replenishes moisture, nourishes the skin, and calms the skin's surface. It will leave your face with a healthy glow. Masks should be applied once a week.

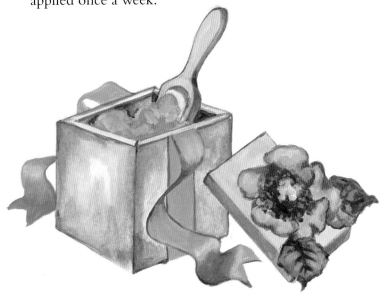

Urban Goddess Facial Mask

Jasmine attracts spiritual love. In India, it is known as "moonlight of the grove." Jasmine warms the emotions and connects us to our more intuitive selves. It is useful for skin of all types.

THE BOTANICALS

1 teaspoon natural yogurt (plain)
2 teaspoons honey
1 vitamin E capsule
1 teaspoon oat flour
5 drops jasmine essential oil

Combine the yogurt and honey. Squeeze the contents of the vitamin E capsule into mixture and stir well. Add oat flour and mix into a smooth paste. Add jasmine essential oil and mix. Apply to face with fingertips. Leave on for 15 minutes, then remove with warm water.

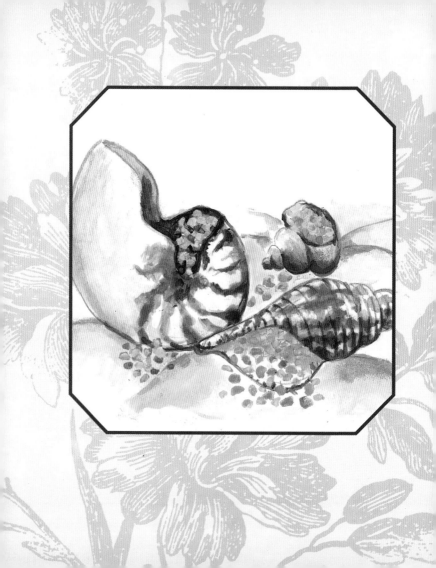

Accouterments
of the Bath

Home Spa Products
and Accessories

Take the time

to come home to yourself everyday.

Robin Casarjean

*F*or a truly indulgent bath and body experience,
the options are limitless. You don't need to go to a spa to
experience thalassotherapy; it is any treatment using
ingredients derived from the sea.

Princess Tremoille's Neroli Salts
For the Royal Bath Treatment

Seventeenth century Princess Tremoille of Nerola was so enamored of the smell of orange blossoms that she used them to scent all that surrounded her. Orange blossom oil became the most sought-after fragrance of the era. To honor her, it was given the name "neroli."

THE BOTANICALS

6-10 drops neroli essential oil
1 teaspoon baking soda
2 teaspoons Epsom salt
3 teaspoons Dead Sea salt

Mix well. Add up to 1/2 cup to hot bath water. Soak 20 minutes.

Salt glow exfoliations and marine algae masks for the entire body can be easily applied at home. Pre-mixed sea-scrubs consisting of mineral enriched sea salts are available in health food stores or specialty body and bath shops.

These stores stock a variety of restorative products and accessories for the bath. They include the loofah, a sea sponge derived from the gourd family that aids in exfoliation and circulation; it comes in the form of a mitt or pad, and some can be found already infused with essential oils. Another option is a natural fiber washcloth, which can be used with aromatic soaps or gels to provide the ultimate cleansing and exfoliation. Natural bristle brushes, used with soap or as a dry brushing treatment, clean and beautify. Irish linen face and body buffs may be applied to the body for a softer touch.

Useful tools for environmental fragrancing include scented beeswax candles made with essential oils, an electrical diffuser which disperses tiny molecules of essential oils throughout a room, and aromatherapy lamps that use a light bulb or a candle beneath a bowl holding water and aromatic oils.

Art and Love Diffuser Blend
For Honoring What Is Sacred
THE BOTANICALS

15 drops rosewood essential oil
12 drops clary sage essential oil
8 drops helichrysum essential oil
3 drops neroli essential oil

Drop the essential oils into a small glass container with an airtight cover. Combine. Add some of the blend to your diffuser or lamp, as needed.

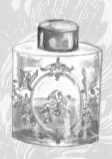

$\mathcal{P}$erfume oil, soap, bath and shower gel, hair products, massage oil, and floral water that use essential oils to scent are recommended for those who do not choose to create their own concoctions. Pure essential oils and candle and aromatherapy kits are the ideal choice for those who do.

However you choose to personalize your bath, always remember that it is for your own pleasure and enjoyment. It is your sacred place to unwind, drift, luxuriate, and heal. Taking a bath is both a fine art and a magical act, a ritual connecting you to all cultures and all times. It is a simple escape from everyday life that promises enduring enchantment.

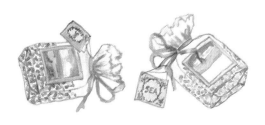

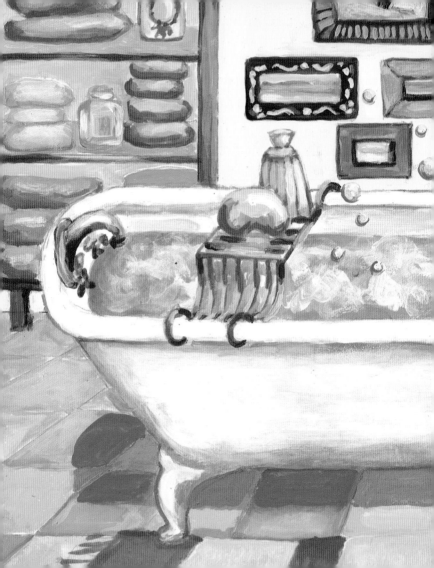

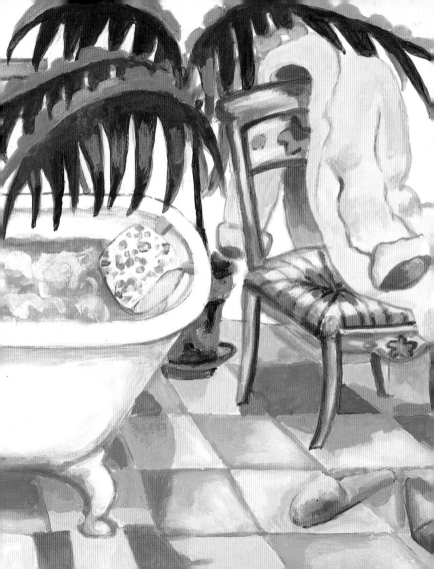

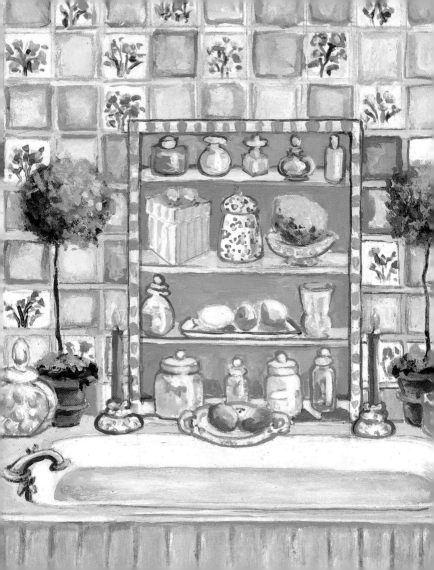